1

Table of Contents

OVERVIEW

High blood sugar (hyperglycemia) affects people who have diabetes. Several factors can contribute to hyperglycemia in people with diabetes, including food and physical activity choices, illness, nondiabetes medications, or skipping or not taking enough glucose-lowering medication.

It's important to treat hyperglycemia, because if left untreated, hyperglycemia can become severe and lead to serious complications requiring emergency care, such as a diabetic coma. In the long term, persistent hyperglycemia, even if not severe, can lead to complications affecting your eyes, kidneys, nerves and heart.

HYPERGLYCEMIA DIET RECIPES

BREAKFAST

1. Mexican Pizza

Prep Time:15 mins

Cook Time: 10 mins

Total Time:25 mins

Servings: 2

Ingredients

- 2 (6 inch) whole-wheat, low carb, tortillas
- 1 egg
- 1 egg whites
- 2 tablespoons canned diced green chiles
- Nonstick cooking spray
- 4 tablespoons bottled salsa
- ¼ cup canned no-salt-added black beans, drained
- 2 tablespoons finely chopped red onion
- 2 tablespoons finely shredded reduced-fat Mexican cheese blend
- ¼ cup chopped avocado

- 2 tablespoons snipped fresh cilantro
- 2 lime wedges

Directions

1. Preheat oven to 400F. Line a baking sheet with foil or parchment paper; set aside.

2. Place tortillas directly onto center oven rack; bake just until crisp, about 4 minutes. Arrange tortillas in a single layer on prepared baking sheet; set aside.

3. In a medium bowl, whisk together the egg, egg white and chiles.

4. Lightly coat a small nonstick skillet with cooking spray. Over medium heat, cook egg mixture, without stirring, until mixture begins to set on the bottom and around edges. With a spatula, lift and fold the partially cooked egg mixture so the uncooked portion flows underneath. Continue cooking 2 to 3 minutes more or until egg mixture is cooked through but is still glossy and moist. Remove from heat and set aside.

5. To assemble pizzas, spread 2 tablespoons salsa over each toasted tortilla. Top with reserved scrambled eggs, black beans, onion and cheese. Bake pizzas on baking sheet 5 to 6 minutes or until heated through.

6. Sprinkle each pizza with avocado and cilantro. Slice into wedges and serve warm with a lime wedge.

2. Meatball Sandwiches

Prep Time:15 Mins

Cook Time: 30 Mins

Total Time: 45 Mins

Serves: 6

Ingredients

Meatballs

- 500 grams beef mince
- 1 small onion, finely chopped
- 1 teaspoon oil
- 1 egg
- ½ teaspoon salt
- ¼ teaspoon pepper
- 2 tablespoons fresh parsley, finely chopped
- ½ teaspoon sage
- ½ teaspoon oregano
- ¼ cup fresh bread crumbs soaked in 2 tablespoons of milk
- ¼ cup panko crumbs
- 2½ cups tomato sauce (your homemade favourite or in a jar from the supermarket)

Sandwiches

- Bread rolls or baguette
- 1 cup Grated Philly & Tasty cheese

Directions:

Meatballs

1. Preheat oven to 180C/350F

2. Sauté onion in a skillet with the oil. Sprinkle a pinch of salt over the onions to help them sweat and not turn brown. Cool.

3. Add all ingredients except sauce to a large mixing bowl and combine with your fingers. Don't overwork and mixture should stay light.

4. Form meatballs and place on a greased baking sheet. Try to make them all the same size so they will cook evenly.

5. Bake for 15 minutes or until the meatballs are nicely browned.

6. Place sauce in a saucepan on medium heat and bring to the boil and then turn down to a bare simmer.

7. When the meatballs are done, add to the sauce.

Sandwiches

1. Cut the bread to make a pocket for and add the meatballs and sauce to the roll. Top with the grated cheese and place in the oven at 180C/350F for about 10 minutes or until the cheese begins to turn a golden brown on the edges.

3. Stuffed French Toast

Prep :5 mins

Cook Time: 20 mins

Total Time :25 mins

Servings: 8

Ingredients

- ½ cup fat-free cream cheese (about 5 ounces)
- 2 tablespoons strawberry or apricot spreadable fruit
- 8 1-inch slices French bread
- 2 egg whites
- 1 egg, slightly beaten
- ¾ cup fat-free milk
- ½ teaspoon vanilla
- ⅛ teaspoon apple pie spice
- Nonstick cooking spray
- ½ cup strawberry or apricot spreadable fruit

Directions:

1. In small bowl, combine cream cheese and 2 tablespoons spreadable fruit. Using serrated knife, form pocket in each bread slice by making a

horizontal cut halfway between top and bottom crust, slicing not quite all the way through. Fill each pocket with about 1 tablespoon of the cream cheese mixture.

2. In small bowl, combine egg whites, egg, milk, vanilla and apple pie spice. Lightly coat nonstick griddle with cooking spray; heat over medium heat.

3. Dip stuffed bread slices into egg mixture, coating both sides. Place bread slices on hot griddle. Cook about 3 minutes or until golden brown, turning once.

4. Meanwhile, in small saucepan, heat 1/2 cup spreadable fruit until melted, stirring frequently. Serve over French toast.

4. California-Style Sandwich

Prep Time:10 mins

Cook Time: 10 mins

Total Time:20 mins

Servings:1

Ingredients

- 1 tablespoon roasted garlic avocado-oil mayonnaise
- 1 everything bagel thin, toasted
- 1 slice Monterey Jack cheese
- ¼ avocado, sliced
- 2 tablespoons alfalfa sprouts
- 1 large egg, fried
- 2 tablespoons thinly sliced red onion

Directions:

1. Spread mayonnaise on 1 bagel thin half. Top with cheese, avocado, sprouts, fried egg and onion. Top with the remaining bagel thin half.

5. Huevos Rancheros Nachos

Prep :20 mins

Cook Time: 10 mins

Total Time :30 mins

Servings:4

Ingredients

- 4 ½ cups baked tortilla chips (3 ounces)
- ¼ teaspoon cumin seeds
- ½ cup canned black beans, rinsed and drained
- ½ cup bottled salsa
- 2 eggs
- 3 egg whites
- 3 tablespoons fat-free milk
- ⅛ teaspoon ground black pepper
- Nonstick cooking spray
- ½ cup shredded reduced-fat Mexican cheese blend (2 ounces)

Directions:

1. Divide chips among serving plates, spreading into single layers; set aside. In a dry small saucepan, heat

cumin seeds over medium heat about 1 minute or until aromatic, stirring frequently. Stir in black beans and salsa. Cook for 1 to 2 minutes or until heated through, stirring occasionally. Remove from heat; cover and keep warm.

2. In a medium bowl, whisk together eggs, egg whites, milk, and pepper. Coat a medium nonstick skillet with cooking spray; heat skillet over medium heat. Pour in egg mixture. Cook over medium heat, without stirring, until mixture starts to set on the bottom and around edge. Using a spatula or a large spoon, lift and fold the partially cooked egg mixture so that the uncooked portion flows underneath. Continue cooking for 2 to 3 minutes or until egg mixture is cooked through, but is still glossy and moist. Remove from heat immediately.

3. Break up cooked eggs and spoon onto tortilla chips. Top with salsa mixture and cheese. Serve immediately.

6. Egg-Stuffed Potatoes

Prep Time:25 mins

Cook Time: 20 mins

Total Time:45 mins

Servings:6

Ingredients

- 3 small-to-medium russet potatoes (6-8 ounces each)
- 2 tablespoons butter
- ½ cup finely chopped red bell pepper
- ¼ cup sliced scallions
- 3 large eggs, beaten
- ¼ teaspoon salt
- ¼ teaspoon ground pepper
- ½ cup shredded Mexican cheese blend

Directions:

1. Prick potatoes with a fork in several places. Microwave on High for 5 minutes. Turnover and continue cooking on High until tender all the way through, about 4 minutes more. (Alternatively, bake at 350 degrees F until tender, 50 minutes to 1 hour.) When cool enough to handle, cut the potatoes in half

lengthwise and scoop out the flesh, leaving a 1/4-inch border. Chop enough of the potato flesh to equal about 1 cup. (Save the remaining potato for another use or discard.)

2. Heat butter in a large nonstick skillet over medium-high heat. Add bell pepper, scallions and the chopped potato. Cook, stirring often, until the pepper softens, 3 to 4 minutes. Add eggs, salt and pepper and cook, stirring, until set, 1 to 2 minutes. Remove from heat. Fold in cheese.

3. Generously stuff each potato half with about 1/2 cup of the egg mixture. Let cool completely, then individually wrap with heavy-duty foil. Refrigerate or store in a cold cooler for up to 1 day.

4. Prepare a campfire and let it burn down to the coals. Place the wrapped potato boats 4 to 6 inches above the coals; cook, turning once or twice, until steaming hot and completely heated through, 10 to 15 minutes. Open carefully. (Alternatively, unwrap and reheat in the microwave.)

7. Egg and Potato

Prep :20 mins

Cook Time:15 mins

Total Time:25 mins

Servings:1

Ingredients

- 5 to 6 spears of cooked asparagus
- 1 tomato, diced
- ¾ cup egg substitute, cooked and scrambled
- ½ cup boiled or roasted yellow potatoes, halved or quartered
- 1 cup honeydew melon (Optional)
- ⅔ cup fat-free yogurt (Optional)

Directions:

1. Arrange cooked asparagus and diced tomato onto one half of a plate. On the other half of the plate place the cooked scrambled eggs and yellow potatoes.
2. Serve with honeydew and yogurt to complete this balanced meal.

8. Christmas Casserole

Prep:20 mins

Cook Time: 1 hr 10 mins

Total Time:1 hr 30 mins

Servings:8

Ingredients

- 1 (10 ounce) package frozen chopped spinach, thawed
- 1 (9 ounce) box frozen artichoke hearts, thawed
- ¾ cup chopped sun-dried tomatoes
- 1 tablespoon extra-virgin olive oil
- 2 cloves garlic, finely chopped
- ½ teaspoon crushed red pepper
- 1 teaspoon lemon zest
- 2 cups low-fat milk
- 5 large eggs
- 1 cup crumbled feta cheese
- 12 ounces rustic whole-wheat bread, torn into 1-inch pieces (about 8 cups

Directions:

1. Place spinach in a clean kitchen towel and squeeze firmly over the sink to remove as much liquid as possible. Combine the squeezed spinach and artichoke hearts in a medium bowl.

2. Cook tomatoes, oil, garlic, crushed red pepper and lemon zest in a small skillet over low heat, stirring often, until fragrant and the garlic is golden brown, 3 to 4 minutes. Stir into the spinach mixture.

3. Preheat oven to 350 degrees F.

4. Whisk milk and eggs in a large bowl. Add the spinach mixture, feta and bread. Toss gently until the bread absorbs the milk mixture. Spoon the mixture into a 13-by-9-inch glass or ceramic baking dish. Let stand at room temperature for 20 to 30 minutes.

5. Bake until set and browned in spots, about 35 minutes. Let stand for 5 to 10 minutes before serving.

9. Toasted Apple-Cheese Sandwiches

Prep Time:10 mins

Cook Tme: 20 mins

Total Time:30 mins

Servings:4

Ingredients

- 1 pound Rome, Braeburn, Golden Delicious and/or Jonathan apples (3 medium), quartered, cored and thinly sliced
- 2 tablespoons water
- ¼ teaspoon ground allspice
- ⅓ cup tub-style light cream cheese, softened
- 2 ounces white cheddar cheese, shredded (1/2 cup)
- 2 oval multi-grain wraps
- ¼ cup chopped walnuts or slivered almonds, toasted

Directions:

1. In a large skillet, combine apple slices, the water and allspice. Cook, covered, over medium heat about 6 minutes or just until apples are tender, stirring occasionally. Uncover; cook about 1 minute more or until liquid is evaporated. Spread cream cheese over

wraps, leaving a 1/2-inch border around the edges. Top one half of each wrap with apple mixture. Sprinkle with white cheddar cheese and walnuts. Fold in half. Lightly coat the tops of the wraps with nonstick spray.

2. Heat a 12-inch nonstick skillet or griddle over medium heat. Add wraps to the skillet, coated sides down. Coat tops of wraps with nonstick spray. Cook for 6 to 10 minutes or until lightly browned, turning once to brown both sides evenly.

3. Cut into wedges to serve.

10. Bacon-Cheese Casserole

Prep :35 mins

Cook Time: 3 hrs 25 mins

Total Time :4 hrs

Servings:8

Ingredients

- 6 light multi-grain English muffins, cut into 1-inch pieces
- Disposable slow cooker liner
- Nonstick cooking spray
- 1 (12 ounce) package (18 slices) lower-sodium less-fat bacon, crisp-cooked, drained and coarsely chopped
- ½ medium zucchini, halved lengthwise and sliced (1 cup)
- ½ cup chopped onion (1 medium)
- ½ cup bottle roasted red sweet pepper, coarsely chopped
- 3 ounces Gouda cheese, shredded (3/4 cup), divided
- ¼ cup finely shredded Parmesan cheese (about 1 ounce)
- 2 cups fat-free milk

- 1 cup refrigerated or frozen egg product, thawed if frozen
- ¼ teaspoon salt
- ¼ teaspoon black pepper

Directions:

1. Preheat oven to 350 degrees F. Spread English muffin pieces in a 15x10x1-inch baking pan. Bake for 10 to 12 minutes or until dried. Remove from oven and cool. Meanwhile, line the removable crockery liner of a 4-quart slow cooker with a disposable slow cooker liner; coat with cooking spray; set aside.

2. In a very large bowl toss together the bread cubes, bacon, zucchini, onion, roasted red pepper, 1/2 cup of the Gouda and the Parmesan. Spoon mixture into the prepared cooker. In the same bowl whisk together milk, egg product, salt and pepper. Pour egg mixture over bread mixture in cooker. Press lightly with the back of a spoon to moisten bread completely.

3. Place crockery liner in the slow cooker. Cover and cook on low-heat setting for 3 to 3 1/2 hours or until an instant-read thermometer registers 200 degrees F

to 210 degrees F when inserted in the center of the casserole. To ensure even cooking, carefully rotate crockery liner 180 degrees halfway through cooking, if possible. Turn off cooker. Remove crockery liner from cooker. Sprinkle remaining 1/4 cup Gouda over casserole. Let stand 30 minutes before serving.

LUNCH

11. Tijuana Torta

Prep Time: 5 mins

Cook Time: 15 mins

Total Time: 20 mins

Ingredients

- 1 15-ounce can black beans, or pinto beans, rinsed (see Note)
- 3 tablespoons prepared salsa
- 1 tablespoon chopped pickled jalapeño
- ½ teaspoon ground cumin
- 1 ripe avocado, pitted
- 2 tablespoons minced onion
- 1 tablespoon lime juice
- 1 16- to 20-inch-long baguette, preferably whole-grain
- 1 ⅓ cups shredded green cabbage

Directions:

1. Mash beans, salsa, jalapeno and cumin in a small bowl. Mash avocado, onion and lime juice in another small bowl.

2. Cut baguette into 4 equal lengths. Split each piece in half horizontally. Pull out most of the soft bread from the center so you're left with mostly crust. Divide the bean paste, avocado mixture and cabbage evenly among the sandwiches. Cut each in half and serve.

12. Italian Vegetable Hoagies

Prep Time:5 mins

Cook Time: 15 mins

Total Time: 20 mins

Servings:4

Ingredients

- 1/4 cup thinly sliced red onion, separated into rings
- 1 14-ounce can artichoke hearts, rinsed and coarsely chopped
- 1 medium tomato, seeded and diced
- 2 tablespoons balsamic vinegar
- 1 tablespoon extra-virgin olive oil
- 1 teaspoon dried oregano
- 1 16- to 20-inch-long baguette, preferably whole-grain
- 2 slices provolone cheese, (about 2 ounces), halved
- 2 cups shredded romaine lettuce
- 1/4 cup sliced pepperoncini, (optional)

Directions

1. Place onion rings in a small bowl and add cold water to cover. Set aside while you prepare the remaining ingredients.

2. Combine artichoke hearts, tomato, vinegar, oil and oregano in a medium bowl. Cut baguette into 4 equal lengths. Split each piece horizontally and pull out about half of the soft bread from each side. Drain the onions and pat dry.

3. To assemble sandwiches, divide provolone among the bottom pieces of baguette. Spread on the artichoke mixture and top with the onion, lettuce and pepperoncini, if using. Cover with the baguette tops. Serve immediately.

13. Creamy Avocado & White Bean Wrap

Prep :10 mins

Cook Time: 15 mins

Total Time: 25 mins

Servings:4

Ingredients

- 2 tablespoons cider vinegar
- 1 tablespoon canola oil
- 2 teaspoons finely chopped canned chipotle chile in adobo sauce, (see Note)
- ¼ teaspoon salt
- 2 cups shredded red cabbage
- 1 medium carrot, shredded
- ¼ cup chopped fresh cilantro
- 1 15-ounce can white beans, rinsed
- 1 ripe avocado
- ½ cup shredded sharp Cheddar cheese
- 2 tablespoons minced red onion
- 4 8- to 10-inch whole-wheat wraps, or tortillas

Directions

1. Whisk vinegar, oil, chipotle chile and salt in a medium bowl. Add cabbage, carrot and cilantro; toss to combine.

2. Mash beans and avocado in another medium bowl with a potato masher or fork. Stir in cheese and onion.

3. To assemble the wraps, spread about 1/2 cup of the bean-avocado mixture onto a wrap (or tortilla) and top with about 2/3 cup of the cabbage-carrot slaw. Roll up. Repeat with remaining ingredients. Cut the wraps in half to serve, if desired.

14. Chipotle-Orange Broccoli & Tofu

Prep Time:10 mins

Cook Time: 20 mins

Total Time: 30 mins

Servings:4

Ingredients

- 1 14-ounce package extra-firm water-packed tofu
- ½ teaspoon salt, divided
- 3 tablespoons canola oil, divided
- 6 cups broccoli florets
- 1 cup orange juice
- 1 tablespoon minced chipotle in adobo (see Tip), seeded if desired
- ½ cup chopped fresh cilantro

Directions

1. Drain tofu and pat dry; cut into 1/2- to 3/4-inch cubes. Sprinkle tofu on all sides with 1/4 teaspoon salt. Heat 2 tablespoons oil in a large nonstick skillet over medium-high heat. Add tofu and cook in a single layer, stirring every couple of minutes, until golden brown, 7 to 9 minutes total. Transfer to a plate.

2. Add the remaining 1 tablespoon oil and broccoli to the pan and sprinkle with the remaining 1/4 teaspoon salt; cook, stirring, until the broccoli is bright green, about 1 minute. Add orange juice and chipotle and cook, stirring frequently, until the broccoli is just tender, 2 to 3 minutes more.

3. Return the tofu to the pan. Cook, gently stirring, until the tofu is heated through, 1 to 2 minutes. Remove from the heat and stir in cilantro.

15. Baked Stuffed Mushrooms

Prep Time:15 Mins

Cook Time:25 Mins

Total Time:40 Mins

Serves: 4

Ingredients

- Buttered Bread Crumbs
- 4 slices of bread processed into fine crumbs in food processor
- 2 tbs butter

Mushroom Stuffing

- 1 lb. button mushrooms, wiped clean and chopped and the stems from the large mushrooms (I used the food processor)
- 1 tablespoon ricotta cheese
- ¼ cup freshly grated parmesan cheese
- 2 tbs butter
- ¼ cup finely chopped onion
- 1 clove garlic finely minced
- 2 slices bacon, chopped into small pieces

- ½ tsp salt

- Black pepper to taste

- 2 tbs grated carrot

- 1 tbs olive oil

- ½ tsp mixed herbs

Stuffed Mushrooms

- 8 large portobello or field mushrooms, cleaned or peeled, stems removed

Directions

1. In a frying pan, saute bacon pieces for a few minutes and then add the carrot and onions with a little bit of salt and cook for 2 minutes.

2. Add the mushrooms and butter and cook on medium high heat for 2 minutes and then add the garlic and cook for a minute or so longer. Set aside to cool in a bowl.

3. In the same frying pan melt 2 tbs butter and when it begins to foam add the bread crumbs and stir to coat. Do not let them turn brown - the oven will do that bit.

4. To the bowl with the mushroom mixture add the ricotta cheese, parmesan cheese, remainder of the salt, some black pepper and the mixed herbs and stir to combine.

5. With a pastry brush, spread oil over the top and bottom of the large mushrooms and place cavity side up in a greased baking pan. (I used spray oil but you could use baking paper)

6. Divide the mushroom mixture between the mushrooms, piling it in the center.

7. Place in oven for 10 minutes before topping with the buttered bread crumbs and bake for an additional 15 minutes or until the crumbs are golden brown.

8. Garnish with chopped parsley.

16. Eggplant And Caramelized Onion Dip

Prep Time:10 Mins

Cook Time:30 Mins

Total Time:40 Mins

6 Servings:

Ingredients

- 1 large eggplant
- 1 cup caramelized onions
- ¼ cup Greek Yogurt
- ⅛ teaspoon ground cumin
- ⅛ teaspoon ground coriander
- ⅛ teaspoon salt (or to taste)
- a few grinds of fresh black pepper

Directions

1. In the BBQ or in the oven, roast the eggplant on high until the insides soften. I left mine in the BBQ for about 30 minutes but watch it. Temperatures might be different.

2. Let cool.

3. Add the caramelized onions to the blender and whiz for a few seconds. You want them broken up but not paste.

4. Scrape the eggplant pulp into a blender

5. Add remaining ingredients and whiz just to combine into a dip. I left mine just a bit lumpy.

6. Place in serving bowl and drizzle with good olive oil and a dusting of paprika.

17. Puff Pastry Tarts

Prep Time:15 Mins

Cook Time:25 Mins

Total Time:40 Mins

Servings: 4

Ingredients

- 1 sheet frozen puff pastry
- 4 eggs
- ½ onion chopped
- 2 slices bacon, chopped
- ¼ cup cheese, (cheddar, mixture, gruyere anything you like or no cheese)
- salt and pepper
- 1 tablespoon chopped parsley

Directions

1. Preheat oven to 200C/400F

2. Cut thawed pastry into 4 squares using a pizza cutter or knife but if you use a knife, don't drag it through the pastry, straight cut down so the pastry will puff up properly.

3. Place each square in the bottom of a cupcake tin. I used 4 corner positions and left the corners sticking out of the cup. Cover with plastic wrap and place in the refrigerator until needed.

4. Saute bacon until nearly crispy and set aside.

5. Saute onion in the bacon fat until translucent.

6. Take the pastry from the refrigerator and place a bit of bacon, onion and cheese on the bottom and crack an egg on top. Sprinkle with salt and pepper and into the oven for 20-25 minutes until the egg is cooked and the pastry is golden brown.

18. Cinnamon Rolls

Prep Time:1 Hour 15 Mins

Cook Time:15 Mins

Total Time:1 Hour 30 Mins

Servings: 12

Ingredients

Dough

- 240 grams milk
- 65 grams Butter
- 2 eggs
- 1 teaspoon salt
- 650 grams bakers flour
- 100 grams sugar
- 10 grams dry yeast

Filling

- 250 grams brown sugar, to taste dark or light
- 65 grams Butter, room temperature
- 2½ tablespoons cinnamon

Icing

- 250 grams raw sugar

- 55 grams Butter

- 125 grams cream cheese

- 1 centimetre vanilla bean

- ⅛ teaspoon salt

Directions

Dough

1. Weigh milk and butter into TM mixing bowl. Heat on 50 degrees C for 3 min on speed 1.

2. Add remaining dough ingredients in order given.

3. Process 15 seconds on speed 7 to make a rough dough.

4. Knead 2 minutes on dough mode.

5. Turn dough out onto Thermomat or into a greased bowl and let prove for 1 hour or until doubled.

6. Roll out dough on Thermomat or lightly floured surface to 35 x 50 cm rectangle.

7. Let rest while preparing filling.

Filling

1. Spread dough with softened 65 g butter

2. Sprinkle evenly with brown sugar and cinnamon. (Yes, this is 2½ TABLEspoons This recipe is very caramel-and-cinnamon.

3. Roll dough from long side and cut into 12 rolls

4. Place rolls in a lightly greased 23 x 33 cm baking tin lined with baking paper. Cover and let rise for 30 minutes; meanwhile, preheat your oven to 200C / 400F

5. Bake in a preheated oven for approx 15 minutes, or until golden.

6. While baking, prepare the icing.

Icing

1. Mill sugar together with vanilla bean into icing sugar 20 seconds on speed 9. (substitute ½ teaspoon pure

vanilla paste or extract after milling sugar if you don't have a vanilla bean)

2. Add butter, cream cheese and salt. Heat on 37 degrees for 2 minutes on speed 2.

3. Spread icing on hot rolls

19. Barbecue Chicken Pizza

Prep Time:45 mins

Cook Time: 1 hr

Total Time:1 hr 45 mins

Servings:5

Ingredients

- 1 pound boneless, skinless chicken breast
- ¾ cup barbecue sauce (see Tip)
- 1 pound whole-wheat pizza dough
- 2 tablespoons extra-virgin olive oil, divided
- 1 medium zucchini
- 1 cup shredded part-skim mozzarella cheese
- ¼ cup Chopped fresh parsley or cilantro for garnish

Directions

1. Preheat oven to 425 degrees F. Coat a large rimmed baking sheet with cooking spray.

2. Place chicken in a large saucepan and add water to cover by 2 inches. Bring to a simmer. Reduce heat to maintain a gentle simmer and cook until an instant-

read thermometer inserted into the thickest part of the chicken registers 165 degrees F, about 15 minutes.

3. Remove the chicken to a clean cutting board. (Discard poaching liquid or save for another use.) Let cool slightly, then shred the chicken into bite-size pieces with two forks. Transfer to a bowl and stir in 1/4 cup barbecue sauce.

4. Meanwhile, roll pizza dough out on a lightly floured surface to the approximate size of the baking sheet. Transfer to the prepared baking sheet and brush with 1 tablespoon oil. Bake until golden in spots, about 10 minutes.

5. Grate zucchini through the large holes on a box grater; pat dry with a clean kitchen towel. Combine the zucchini with the remaining 1/2 cup barbecue sauce in a small bowl.

6. Turn the crust over and brush with the remaining 1 tablespoon oil. Evenly top with the saucy zucchini, the chicken and mozzarella. Continue baking until the cheese is melted, 6 to 8 minutes more. Serve sprinkled with parsley (or cilantro), if desired.

20. Apple Bran Muffins

Prep Time:8 Mins

Cook Time:20 Mins

Total Time:28 Mins

Servings: 12

Ingredients

- 1¼ cups all-purpose flour (I sifted the flour, baking powder, cinnamon and salt)
- 1 tsp cinnamon
- ½ cup sugar
- 1 tablespoon baking powder
- ¼ teaspoon salt
- 2 cups Kellogg's All-Bran Original cereal
- 1¼ cups fat-free milk
- 1 egg
- ¼ cup vegetable oil
- 1 apple chopped

Directions

1. Stir together flour, sugar, cinnamon, baking powder and salt. Set aside.

2. In large mixing bowl, combine KELLOGG'S ALL-
   BRAN cereal and milk. Let stand about 2 minutes or
   until cereal softens.

3. Add egg, sugar and oil. Beat well.

4. Add flour mixture, stirring only until combined.

5. Add apple and barely mix through.

6. Portion evenly into twelve muffin pan cups coated
   with cooking spray.

7. Bake at 400° F about 20 minutes or until golden
   brown. Serve warm.

DINNER

21. Kale Salad with Bacon-Blue Cheese Vinaigrette

Prep Time:10 mins

 Cook Time: 20 mins

Total Time: 30 mins

Servings:6

Ingredients

- 1 pound Yukon Gold potatoes, scrubbed, cut into 1-inch chunks
- 3 tablespoons extra-virgin olive oil, divided
- ½ teaspoon dried thyme
- ½ teaspoon salt, divided
- ½ teaspoon freshly ground pepper, divided
- 6 cups kale, stems removed, torn into bite-size pieces
- 3 tablespoons cider vinegar
- 3 tablespoons crumbled blue cheese
- 2 tablespoons minced shallot
- 1 tablespoon honey mustard
- 1 tablespoon minced fresh parsley
- 3 pieces center-cut bacon, cooked and crumbled
- 2 Belgian endives, cored and sliced

- ¼ cup currants or sweetened dried cranberries

Directions

1. Preheat oven to 400 degrees F.

2. Toss potatoes, 1 tablespoon oil, thyme and 1/4 teaspoon each salt and pepper in a large bowl. Spread out on a large baking sheet (reserve the bowl). Roast the potatoes, stirring once or twice, until tender and browned, 15 to 20 minutes.

3. Place kale in the large bowl, add the hot potatoes and let stand for several minutes, tossing occasionally, until the potatoes are warm but not hot.

4. Meanwhile, whisk the remaining 2 tablespoons oil, vinegar, blue cheese, shallot, mustard, parsley and the remaining 1/4 teaspoon salt and pepper in a small bowl.

5 Drizzle the dressing over the warm salad. Add bacon, endive and currants (or cranberries); toss to combine. Serve immediately.

22. Orange & Black Pepper Shrimp Salad

Prep Time:15 mins

Cook Time: 25 mins

Total Time: 40 mins

Servings:4

Ingredients

- 3 medium oranges
- 2 teaspoons whole black peppercorns, divided
- 2 cups loosely packed flat-leaf parsley leaves (about 1 large bunch), divided
- 4 tablespoons chopped toasted walnuts (see Tips), divided
- 3 tablespoons walnut oil, divided
- 2 tablespoons red-wine vinegar
- teaspoons capers, rinsed, divided
- 2 teaspoons Dijon mustard
- 2 teaspoons honey
- 1 small clove garlic, minced
- ¼ teaspoon salt
- 1 large head Treviso or small head radicchio, cut into bite-size pieces

- 1/2 small head romaine or 1 heart of romaine, cut into bite-size pieces
- 3 cups arugula
- 1 pound peeled and deveined raw shrimp (21-25 per pound; see Tips)

Directions

1. With a sharp knife, remove the skin and white pith from oranges. Working over a bowl, cut the segments from their surrounding membranes. Squeeze juice into the bowl before discarding the membranes. Transfer the orange segments to another bowl with a slotted spoon and set aside.

2. Crush peppercorns with a mortar and pestle or place in a small sealable bag and crush with a small heavy skillet, the smooth side of a meat mallet or a rolling pin.

3. Pour 1/4 cup of the orange juice from the bowl into a blender. Add 1/4 teaspoon of the crushed pepper, 1 cup parsley, 3 tablespoons walnuts, 2

tablespoons oil, vinegar, 2 teaspoons capers, mustard, honey, garlic and salt; puree until smooth.

4. Combine Treviso (or radicchio), romaine, arugula and the remaining 1 cup parsley in a large bowl. Toss with 1/2 cup of the dressing.

5. Heat the remaining 1 tablespoon oil in a large nonstick skillet over medium-high heat. Sprinkle shrimp with the remaining crushed pepper. Add the shrimp to the hot skillet and cook until bright pink and browned, 1 to 3 minutes per side.

6. Transfer the salad to a platter or 4 dinner plates. Top with the reserved orange segments, the shrimp and the remaining 4 teaspoons capers and 1 tablespoon walnuts. Serve drizzled with the remaining dressing.

23. Curried Parsnip & Apple Soup

Prep Time:25 mins

Cook Time: 40 mins

Total Time: 1 hrs 5 mins

Servings:4

Ingredients

- 1 tablespoon extra-virgin olive oil
- 1 ½ pounds parsnips (about 5 medium), peeled, cored and chopped
- 1 large onion, finely chopped
- 3 medium cloves garlic, finely chopped
- 4 cups low-sodium chicken broth
- 1 cup water
- 1 medium russet potato (about 8 ounces), peeled and chopped
- 1 large Granny Smith apple, peeled and chopped
- 1 ½ teaspoons mild curry powder
- 1 ½ teaspoons ground coriander, plus more for garnish
- 1 teaspoon ground cumin
- ½ teaspoon ground ginger

- 4 teaspoons lemon juice
- ½ teaspoon salt
- ¼ teaspoon freshly ground pepper
- ½ cup low-fat plain yogurt

Directions

1. Heat oil in a large pot over medium-high heat. Add parsnips and onion and cook, stirring occasionally, until the onion begins to brown, 5 to 7 minutes. Add garlic and cook, stirring occasionally, until fragrant, 45 seconds. Add broth, water, potato, apple, curry powder, coriander, cumin and ginger; bring to a boil. Cover, reduce heat to medium-low and simmer until the vegetables are tender when mashed against the side of the pot with a wooden spoon, about 20 minutes.

2. Puree the soup in the pot with an immersion blender until smooth. (Alternatively, blend the soup in batches in a blender with the lid slightly ajar. Use caution when blending hot liquids. Return the soup to the pot.) Add lemon juice, salt and pepper. Serve with

dollops of yogurt swirled on top, garnished with
pinches of coriander.

24. Savory Cauliflower Cake

Prep Time: 25 mins

Cook Time: 1 hr 20 mins

Total Time: 1hrs 45 mins

Servings:8

Ingredients

- 1 medium head cauliflower (about 2 pounds), trimmed and broken into small florets
- 1 tablespoon extra-virgin olive oil
- 1 medium onion, thinly sliced
- ¾ teaspoon caraway seed, ground or crushed
- ½ teaspoon ground coriander
- ½ teaspoon crushed red pepper, or to taste
- ¾ teaspoon salt, divided
- ¾ cup garbanzo bean flour (see Tip)
- ¼ cup all-purpose flour or gluten-free flour blend
- ½ teaspoon baking powder
- large eggs
- 1 jarred roasted red pepper, rinsed and chopped (about 1/2 cup)
- ¾ cup crumbled feta cheese

- 3 tablespoons chopped fresh dill, divided

Directions

1. Preheat oven to 350 degrees F. Line the bottom and sides of a 9-inch springform pan with parchment paper.

2. Bring about 1 inch of water to a boil in a large pot fitted with a steamer basket. Add cauliflower and steam until tender, 8 to 10 minutes.

3. Heat oil in a large skillet over medium heat. Add onion and cook, stirring, until tender and golden, about 8 minutes. Add caraway seed, coriander, crushed red pepper and 1/2 teaspoon salt; cook, stirring, until fragrant, about 1 minute. Gently stir in the steamed cauliflower, doing your best not to break up the florets, and cook for 2 to 3 minutes to combine the flavors.

4. Whisk garbanzo bean flour, all-purpose flour (or gluten-free blend), baking powder and the remaining 1/4 teaspoon salt in a bowl. Whisk eggs in a large bowl until mixed. Sprinkle the dry

ingredients over the eggs and whisk to combine and eliminate most of the lumps. Stir in roasted red pepper, feta and 2 tablespoons dill. Add the cauliflower mixture and gently stir to combine. Spread the mixture evenly into the prepared pan.

5. Bake until the top is golden and the cake is set, 35 to 45 minutes. Let cool to warm; remove the pan sides and the parchment. Serve warm or at room temperature, garnished with the remaining 1 tablespoon dill.

25. Tilapia Po'Boy

Prep Time: 25 mins

Cook Time: 15 mins

Total Time: 25 mins

Servings:4

Ingredients

- 2 large tilapia fillets (6-7 ounces each)
- 2 teaspoons Cajun spice blend (without added salt)
- ½ teaspoon salt
- 1 large egg white
- 2 tablespoons water
- ½ cup fine cornmeal
- 2 tablespoons canola oil, divided
- 5 tablespoons low-fat mayonnaise
- 3 tablespoons finely chopped dill pickle
- 4 small whole-wheat hoagie buns (2-3 ounces each), toasted
- 2 ripe plum tomatoes, sliced
- ½ cup thinly sliced red onion
- 2 cups very thinly sliced romaine

Directions

1. Sprinkle fish with Cajun spice and salt, then cut each fillet in half lengthwise. Whisk egg white and water in a shallow dish. Place cornmeal in another shallow dish. Dip the fish in the egg mixture, then in the cornmeal. (Discard any leftover egg and cornmeal.)

2. Heat 1 tablespoon oil in a large nonstick skillet over medium-high heat. Add the fish (it will be a tight fit) and cook until golden brown on the bottom, 3 to 5 minutes. Turn over, swirl in the remaining 1 tablespoon oil and cook until the fish is golden brown on the other side and opaque in the middle, 3 to 5 minutes more.

3. Combine mayonnaise and pickle in a small bowl. To assemble the sandwiches, spread 1 generous tablespoon of the mixture on each bun. Top with a piece of fish, tomato, onion and lettuce.

26. Winter Vegetable Dal

Prep Time:15 mins

Cook Time:45 mins

Total Time: 1 hr

Servings:6

Ingredients

- 2 tablespoons coconut oil or canola oil
- 1 teaspoon brown mustard seeds
- 1 teaspoon cumin seeds
- 12 fresh curry leaves (see Tip) or 1 large bay leaf
- 1 medium onion, finely chopped
- 1 serrano chile, finely diced
- 3 tablespoons finely chopped fresh ginger
- 4 medium cloves garlic, finely chopped
- 4 ½ cups water
- 1 ½ cups red lentils (see Tip), rinsed
- 1 (14 ounce) can "lite" coconut milk
- 1 ½ teaspoons salt
- 1 teaspoon ground turmeric
- 2 ½ cups cubed peeled butternut squash
- 2 cups cauliflower florets (1-inch)

- 1 large Yukon Gold potato (about 8 ounces), cut into 1/2-inch chunks
- 1 teaspoon garam masala
- 2 tablespoons lime juice

Directions

1. Heat oil over medium-high heat in a large pot. Add mustard seeds, cumin seeds and curry leaves (if using) and cook until the seeds begin to pop, about 20 seconds. Add onion, chile, ginger and garlic and cook, stirring occasionally, until the onion is starting to brown, about 5 minutes.

2. Add bay leaf (if using), water, lentils, coconut milk, salt and turmeric to the pot. Bring to a boil, stirring frequently to make sure the lentils don't stick to the bottom. Add squash, cauliflower and potato; return to a boil. Reduce heat to a simmer and cook, uncovered, stirring occasionally, until the vegetables are just tender when pierced with a fork, 20 to 25 minutes.

3. Remove from heat; stir in garam masala and lime juice.

27. Oven-Fried Beef Taquitos

Prep Time: 10 mins

Cook Time: 20 mins

Total Time: 30 mins

Servings: 4

Ingredients

- 1 medium zucchini
- 2 teaspoons canola oil
- 1 pound extra-lean ground beef
- 3 tablespoons chili powder
- 2 teaspoons onion powder
- 1 teaspoon ground cumin
- ½ teaspoon salt
- 12 6-inch corn tortillas
- Canola oil cooking spray
- ¾ cup shredded sharp Cheddar cheese

Directions

1. Preheat oven to 425 degrees F.

2. Shred zucchini using the large holes of a box grater. Squeeze dry in a clean kitchen towel (you should have about 2 cups). Heat oil in a large nonstick skillet over medium-high heat. Add the zucchini, beef, chili powder, onion powder, cumin and salt. Cook, stirring, until the beef is cooked through, 5 to 7 minutes

3. Spread tortillas out on a baking sheet in two overlapping rows. Bake until hot, 2 minutes. Transfer to a plate and cover.

4. Coat the baking sheet with cooking spray. Place 6 tortillas on a clean cutting board. Working quickly, spread a generous 1/4 cup beef mixture along the bottom third of a tortilla, sprinkle with about 1 tablespoon cheese and tightly roll into a cigar shape. Place the taquito seam-side down on the baking sheet. Repeat with the remaining tortillas, filling and cheese. Generously coat the top and sides of the taquitos with cooking spray.

5. Bake the taquitos until browned and crispy, 14 to 18 minutes.

28. Indian Saag with Chickpeas

Prep Time:15 mins

Cook Time: 35 mins

Total Time: 50 mins

Servings:4

Ingredients

- ¾ cup brown basmati rice
- 1 ½ cups water
- 2 tablespoons extra-virgin olive oil, divided
- 8 ounces paneer cheese or 16-ounce package water-packed extra-firm tofu, cubed
- 1 small onion, sliced
- 1 15-ounce can chickpeas, rinsed
- 1 tablespoon garam masala
- 2 teaspoons minced fresh ginger
- 2 teaspoons ground cumin
- 10 ounces frozen chopped spinach, thawed
- ¾ cup diced fresh tomatoes or drained canned diced tomatoes
- ½ teaspoon salt
- ½ cup low-fat plain yogurt

Directions

1. Bring rice and water to a boil in a small saucepan. Reduce heat to maintain a low simmer, cover and cook until the rice is tender and the water is absorbed, 30 to 40 minutes (see Tip). Remove from heat and let stand, covered, for 10 minutes. Fluff with a fork.

2. Meanwhile, heat 1 tablespoon oil in a large nonstick skillet over medium-high heat. Add paneer (or tofu) and cook, stirring frequently, until lightly browned, 5 to 10 minutes. Remove to a plate. Reduce the heat to medium and add the remaining 1 tablespoon oil, onion, chickpeas, ginger, garam masala and cumin. Cook, stirring, until the onions are soft, about 10 minutes. Stir in spinach, tomatoes and salt and cook until hot, about 3 minutes. Return the paneer (or tofu) to the pan and cook, gently stirring, until hot, about 1 minute. Remove from heat and stir in yogurt. Serve the rice with the stew.

29. Shrimp, Ham & Pepper Couscous

Prep Time:15 mins

Cook Time: 30 mins

Total Time: 45 mins

Servings:4

Ingredients

Couscous

- 1 tablespoon extra-virgin olive oil
- 3 ounces ham steak, diced
- 1 medium red bell pepper, diced
- 1 small onion, diced
- 3 large cloves garlic, minced
- ½ teaspoon smoked paprika
- ½ teaspoon fennel seed
- ¼ teaspoon salt
- ½ teaspoon ground pepper
- 1 cup no-salt-added diced tomatoes (with juice)
- ¼ cup water
- 1 pound raw shrimp (21-25 per pound), peeled and deveined
- ½ cup frozen peas, thawed

- ½ cup whole-wheat couscous

Salad

- 3 tablespoons extra-virgin olive oil
- 2 tablespoons sherry vinegar
- ⅛ teaspoon salt
- ⅛ teaspoon ground pepper
- 8 cups mixed greens
- ⅓ cup crumbled feta
- ⅓ cup slivered almonds, toasted
- ¼ cup dried cranberries

Directions

1. To prepare couscous: Heat 1 tablespoon oil in a large skillet over medium heat. Add ham, pepper and onion; cook, stirring, until vegetables soften, about 4 minutes. Add garlic, paprika, fennel seed, 1/4 teaspoon salt and 1/2 teaspoon pepper; cook, stirring constantly, until fragrant, about 2 minutes. Stir in tomatoes (with juice) and water. Bring to a simmer; cover and cook for 2 minutes. Stir in shrimp and peas; cook, uncovered and stirring occasionally, until the shrimp are opaque, 2 to 4 minutes. Stir in couscous.

Cover, remove from heat and let stand for 5 minutes; fluff.

2. To prepare salad: Whisk 3 tablespoons oil, vinegar and 1/8 teaspoon each salt and pepper in a large bowl. Add greens; toss to coat with the dressing. Serve topped with almonds, feta and cranberries.

30. Roasted Pepper-&-Cheese Stuffed Chicken

Prep Time:10 mins

Cook Time: 30 mins

Total Time: 40 mins

Servings:4

Ingredients

- ⅓ cup chopped jarred roasted red peppers, rinsed
- ¼ cup shredded provolone cheese
- 2 boneless, skinless chicken breasts (about 1 1/4 pounds), trimmed
- ¾ teaspoon ground pepper, divided
- ½ teaspoon salt
- ½ teaspoon dried oregano
- 2 tablespoons extra-virgin olive oil, divided
- ounces whole-wheat orzo (about 1 cup dry)
- ¼ cup chopped Kalamata olives
- 5 cups broccoli florets
- 2 tablespoons unsalted butter
- 4 lemon wedges, for serving

Directions

1. Preheat oven to 425 degrees F. Coat an 8-inch square baking dish with cooking spray

2. Combine roasted peppers and provolone in a small bowl. Cut a horizontal slit along the thin, long edge of each chicken breast, nearly through to the opposite side. Season the chicken with 1/2 teaspoon pepper, salt and oregano. Fill each chicken breast "pocket" with half of the cheese mixture, and press the edges together to seal. Place the chicken in the prepared baking dish and drizzle with 1 tablespoon oil.

3. Bake the chicken until an instant-read thermometer inserted into the thickest part registers 165 degrees F, 20 to 25 minutes.

4. Meanwhile, cook orzo according to package directions. Drain; transfer to a bowl and toss with olives, the remaining 2 teaspoons oil and 1/4 teaspoon pepper.

5. Steam broccoli over 1 inch of boiling water in a pot fit with a steamer basket until just tender, 4 to 5 minutes. Transfer to a bowl and toss with butter.